Natural & Healthy Sweeteners

Diana Allen, MS, CNS

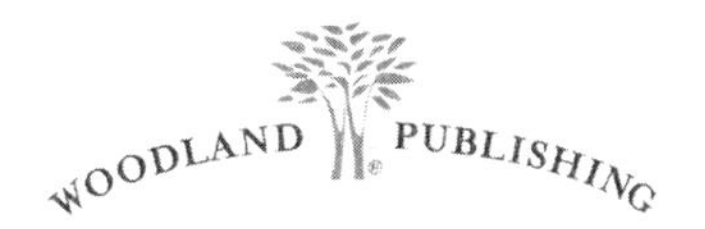

For permissions, ordering information, or bulk quantity discounts, contact:
Woodland Publishing, Salt Lake City, Utah
Visit our Web site: www.woodlandpublishing.com
Toll-free number: (800) 777-BOOK

The information in this book is for educational purposes only and is not recommended as a means of diagnosing or treating an illness. All matters concerning physical and mental health should be supervised by a health practitioner knowledgeable in treating that particular condition. Neither the publisher nor the author directly or indirectly dispenses medical advice, nor do they prescribe any remedies or assume any responsibility for those who choose to treat themselves.

Cataloging-in-Publication data is available from the Library of Congress.

ISBN: 978-1-58054-185-5

Printed in the United States of America

Contents

Part 1: Understanding Sugars and Sweeteners

Part 2: Natural and Healthy Sweeteners

Part 1

Understanding Sugars and Sweeteners

It's Natural to Like Sweets

There's no need to feel guilty if you have a sweet tooth. Most animals actively seek out foods that are sweet tasting, and humans are no exception. Our preference for sweet foods begins at birth and appears to be biologically hardwired right into our DNA, most probably as a survival mechanism that operates on multiple levels.

One of the first things every baby does after leaving the womb and entering the world is to consume food in the form of milk. Milk is sweet. Being held in our mother's arms as this sweet, life-giving liquid fills our tiny mouths and empty bellies is our earliest experience, so it's no wonder we associate the taste of sweetness with feelings of comfort, safety and security.

About seven percent of breast milk is made up of energy-providing carbohydrate sugars, primarily in the form of lactose (also known as milk sugar). Lactose gives milk a light, natural sweetness. And because carbohydrates are the primary energy source for most body organs and tissues, including muscle and brain cells, lactose supports infant growth and development.

Lactose and all sugars, including most natural and healthy sweeteners, are dietary carbohydrates. The following explains a little about what carbohydrates and sugars are and how they function in the body.

Carbohydrates and Sugars: Needed for Life

Many people are most familiar with carbohydrates in relation to the phenomenon of low-carb diets, a popular weight-loss system that, unfortunately, may mistakenly give followers the impression that all carbohydrates are fattening or unhealthy. Nothing could be further from the truth.

With the exception of water, carbohydrates are the largest and most important nutritive component of the human diet. The brain is fueled exclusively by carbohydrates, and most of our energy needs are supplied by carbohydrates. Simply put, people need carbohydrates to live. When it comes to nutrition, health and body weight, what matters is not just the total carbohydrate content of a food but the *type* of carbohydrate a food contains. In general, the "bad guys" are refined and processed carbohydrates, and the "good guys" are whole, natural and complex carbohydrates. To understand why, let's review some quick and easy carbohydrate chemistry.

Meet Your Sugars

Carbohydrates are composed of different types and sizes of sugar molecules. These different sugars (saccharides) are classified into four major groups according to the type and number of sugar units they contain. All sugars are made from three basic elements: carbon, hydrogen and oxygen.

Monosaccharides are the simplest sugars, composed of just one sugar unit per molecule. (The prefix *mono-* means "one.") A monosaccharide sugar unit contain six carbon atoms, 12 hydrogen atoms and six oxygen atoms, giving it the chemical name $C_6H_{12}O_6$. (Because water, or H_2O, also contains hydrogen and oxygen in a 2:1 ratio, it was once thought that carbohydrates were simply hydrated carbon atoms, hence their name.)

Three important monosaccharides are glucose, fructose and galactose. These monosaccharides may exist alone or they may combine to form more complex sugars. Glucose and fructose are very important to the study of natural and healthy sweeteners. Galactose is found in milk, where it is bonded to glucose to form the disaccharide lactose.

Glucose is the most critical sugar for human life and the sugar that is measured to determine blood sugar levels. Glucose is the primary fuel used to make ATP, the energy currency of the body. It is also the primary fuel source for brain and muscle function. Glucose is so important to our bodies that when dietary glucose is not available, we manufacture our own glucose—from noncarbohydrate substrates such as amino acids, lactic acid and glycerol.

Fructose is the sweetest naturally occurring sugar, far sweeter than glucose. Unlike glucose, fructose has a very mild, insignificant impact on blood sugar levels. Fructose is sometimes called fruit sugar because in nature, fructose is found abundantly in fruits and honey, always along with other sugars. Fructose contributes 42 to 55 percent of the sugars in bananas, oranges and grapes, 48 percent of the sugars in honey (on average) and 56 to 65 percent of the sugars in apples, berries and watermelon. Fruit sugar plays interesting roles in the body. Research at the Linus Pauling Institute suggests that when we eat an apple, for example, the fructose it contains may be required to unlock the benefits of antioxidants also present in the fruit.

Disaccharides are double sugars. They consist of two monosaccharide units fused together by a chemical bond. (The prefix *di-* means "two.") Different monosaccharide combinations create the different disaccharides. The most important dietary disaccharides are sucrose, maltose and lactose. Sucrose (table sugar) is a 50-50 blend of glucose and fructose. Each sucrose molecule contains one fructose molecule and one glucose molecule.

Oligosaccharides are sugars composed of three or four monosaccharide sugar units fused together by chemical bonds. (The prefix *oligo-* means "a few.") Found abundantly in legumes and the soluble fiber inulin, oligosaccharides are highly resistant to the action of normal digestive enzymes. This is one reason why beans are notoriously hard to digest for many people. Oligosaccharides are partly digested in the large intestine by gas-producing bacteria through a process called fermentation, which can lead to bloating and flatulence. (The good news is that some by-products of colonic microflora fermentation are health promoting.)

Polysaccharides are the longest type of sugars. (The prefix *poly-* means "many.") Polysaccharides consist of chains of glucose molecules—from dozens to hundreds of glucose units—linked together in straight or branched formation. Amyloses are polysaccharides that display straight-chain formation; branched-chain polysaccharides are called amylopectins. Often, the two are found together in food, notably starches.

Fiber is rich in polysaccharides. Complex carbohydrates contain insoluble fiber (roughage, cellulose) and soluble fiber (pectin, gums) made from amylose, amylopectin and other compounds such as lignans that, like oligosaccharides, also resist digestion. In general, complex carbohydrates containing fiber take several hours to break down in the body, so they have far less impact on blood sugar levels than simple carbohydrates like sucrose that are absorbed very rapidly.

Digestion and Assimilation of Carbohydrates and Sugars

The carbohydrate digestive process splits chemical bonds and turns complex carbs into simple sugars that can be absorbed in the intestines. The rate of absorption varies, depending on the type of carbohydrate or sugar consumed.

The simple sugars found in most sweet and refined or processed carbohydrate-rich foods require short work on the part of the digestive system, making their absorption almost instantaneous. The complex sugars found in natural, fiber-containing carbohydrate sources such as whole grains or sweet potatoes require longer digestion time. As the body breaks apart long-chain starch polysaccharides, glucose molecules are slowly released for absorption.

After glucose is absorbed through the intestinal lining, it travels to the liver and enters the bloodstream. When blood glucose levels increase, a signal is sent to the pancreas to release insulin. Insulin is a hormone that enables glucose to enter cells for energy production. If cells don't need more energy, insulin tells the adipose tissue to store the glucose as fat for later use. In general, the more glucose, and hence insulin, in the system, the more fat that is produced.

Insulin Keeps Blood Sugar in Check

The amount of glucose in the blood is tightly regulated by the insulin response. The job of insulin is to remove glucose from the blood and into the cells as quickly as possible, because the body does not like to have too much glucose in the blood at one time. Healthy blood glucose levels are maintained in the range of 70 to 140 mg/dL (milligrams per deciliter). The higher the blood sugar level rises, the more insulin the pancreas will release to help move glucose out of the blood and keep levels in the healthy range.

Unfortunately, and for reasons not yet well understood, repeatedly flooding the body with too much sugar can cause cells to become resistant to the action of insulin, leading to chronically elevated insulin and blood sugar levels. Insulin resistance may signal the onset of a host of health problems beginning with stubborn weight gain—especially in the abdominal area—and ongoing systemic inflammation. Insulin resistance, when combined with factors such as high abdominal fat, high blood pressure and high cholesterol, is considered a precursor of type 2 diabetes and cardiovascular disease. (Fortunately, it is usually reversible through diet, exercise and stress reduction. Nutritional supplements can also help.)

Keeping blood sugar stable is an important step in helping to maintain a healthy insulin response. Blood sugar balance is also key to avoiding the mood swings, behavioral changes and energy fluctuations—the highs and lows—often associated with sugar consumption. Low glycemic sweeteners can play a role in helping to support healthy blood sugar levels.

The Glycemic Index

Because the body absorbs different types of carbohydrates at different speeds, it makes sense that different types of carbs will raise blood glucose levels at different rates. Not surprisingly, pure glucose is among the fastest at raising blood glucose levels. Scientists used this fact to develop the glycemic index (GI), a system that ranks the effects of various carbohydrate-containing foods on blood sugar levels.

Here's how it works. The GI assigns a value of 100 to the rate at which 50 grams of pure glucose raises blood sugar levels in one or two hours. (A test subject's blood sugar level is tested before and after consuming the glucose.) The result is given the value of 100. Other single foods are then tested in the same way, again in 50 gram amounts. A GI value is assigned to each food depending on how quickly it raises the blood sugar relative to the reference point of 100 for pure glucose. The faster a food raises blood sugar levels relative to the glucose rate, the higher it will rank on the glycemic index scale. (Note: A different GI scale based on 50 grams of white bread to set the benchmark value of 100 is also in use. This can be confusing. GI tables should specify whether the values listed are relative to glucose or white bread.)

Low vs. High Glycemic Foods

A food is considered to be high glycemic if it ranks at or above 70 on the glycemic index scale. Foods ranking between 69 and 55 are considered moderate glycemic, and those below 55 are considered low glycemic foods.

Low glycemic foods typically contain more water, fiber, fat or protein than high glycemic foods. Hence legumes, nuts and dairy products are typically low glycemic, as are most fresh vegetables and tart fruits such as berries and grapefruit. Baked goods (bread, crackers, cookies), grains and sugar-sweetened foods (soft drinks, energy drinks, candy bars) are typically high glycemic.

There are some interesting surprises in the GI table. The glycemic index of pasta is relatively low (30 to 60), even though it is a refined/processed carbohydrate. This is probably due to the way starch and gluten molecules interact in the spongelike matrix of pasta dough.

Another surprise is that the very low GI of some raw fruits and vegetables increases when these foods are cooked. For instance, raw carrots and corn are lower glycemic than cooked carrots and corn.

Also, the glycemic index of some cooked vegetables changes with the variety and mode of preparation (e.g., baking vs. boiling). For example, the GI of white potatoes may range 40 points or more, from 54 for a boiled Canadian spud to 94 and up for an American baked Russet. Sometimes, a food's GI depends upon its temperature when eaten, making it impossible to assign an exact, unchanging value to many food items.

To further complicate things, consider that in practice, nobody eats exactly 50 gram portions of single foods in isolation, the standard measure and protocol for determining GI values. To help address this fact, a "sister" scale called the glycemic load (GL) was developed. Unlike the GI, the GL bases values on the total grams of carbohydrate found in an average portion size of any given item, such as one five gram teaspoon of jam rather than a massive 50 grams, the amount used in the GI.

It's useful to gain a basic familiarity with GI and GL values, especially if you are dealing with overweight or blood sugar issues. A complete international table of glycemic index and glycemic load values for hundreds of food items was compiled in 2002 and published in the *American Journal of Clinical Nutrition*. The table, which includes a wide variety of branded products and numerous traditional foods from around the world, may be viewed online.

Bringing Home the GI Message

As valuable as the glycemic index is, in real life people eat varying portion sizes of foods in various combinations. That five grams of jam is more likely to find itself spread with peanut butter between two slices of bread than flying solo on a lonely teaspoon. Hence the actual speed at which your blood sugar level will rise following consumption of a peanut butter and jelly sandwich, or any meal, depends on how long it takes to digest and absorb all the sugars contained therein.

It is impossible to determine a GI value for every meal you might ever consume. Luckily, there's no real need for this information because, specific values aside, the take-home message is simple: Base your diet on low glycemic foods that help to keep your blood sugar levels balanced and stable. Research strongly suggests that high glycemic diets, when eaten over the long term, may contribute to a variety of health problems, including obesity and increased risk for type 2 diabetes, cardiovascular disease and some cancers.

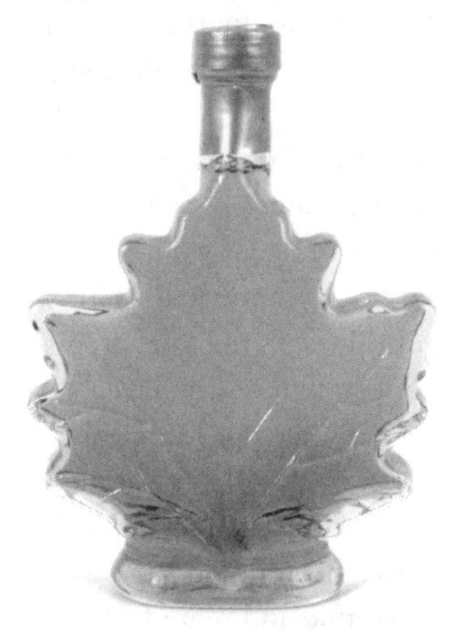

Maple syrup is considered low on the glycemic index.

Low glycemic diets that include abundant amounts of fresh vegetables and high-fiber whole foods, moderate amounts of fresh fruit and recommended levels of healthy fats and proteins are best. And when it's time for dessert, consider treats made with low glycemic natural and healthy sweeteners.

It is no coincidence that most low glycemic foods are high in micronutrients and other beneficial compounds. Impact on blood sugar levels is important, but it is not the sole measure of the healthfulness or harmfulness of any food or sweetener. To determine which foods and sweeteners are most appropriate for you, consider your personal health goals and biochemically individual needs along with factors such as nutrient density (vitamin, mineral and macronutrient content); energy potential (caloric value); antioxidant and phytonutrient content; anti-nutrient content, if any (e.g., phytates, oxalates); hydrating properties (water content); sodium content; enzyme content; presence of harmful substances (e.g., chlorine, aluminum, synthetic preservatives); and subtle features such as the vitality or amount of life-force energy.

The following table provides glycemic index values for some of the sweeteners discussed in this booklet.

Table 1
Glycemic Index of Selected Sugars and Sweeteners

Sweetener	Glycemic index
Erythritol	0
Stevia	<1
Artificial sweeteners	<1
Xylitol	8
Fructose	19
Raw honey*	32–58
Agave syrup*	30–40
Palm sugar	35
Maltitol (crystalline)	36
Maple syrup	54
Blackstrap molasses	55
Pasteurized honey*	62–87
Sucrose (table sugar)	68
Corn syrup	75
High fructose corn syrup	87
Glucose	100

* GI varies with species, variety or production method.

Note: Values below 55 are considered low glycemic; values between 55 and 69 are considered moderate glycemic; values of 70 and above are considered high glycemic.

Sources: www.ajcn.org/cgi/content/full/76/1/5/T1; www.glycemicindex.com/

The Brain-Sugar Connection

Food exerts tremendous power throughout our lives by its association with events integrated into memory. I can remember being a little girl and returning home with my father from ice skating at the local pond. Once I'd wriggled out from all the layers of winter gear, Dad made me a mug of hot cocoa with marshmallows, which I savored with delight. Many years have since passed, but I can still remember how the first sip of that piping hot elixir burned the tip of my tongue, taste the richness of the liquid chocolate and clearly conjure the soft squish of marshmallows melting in my mouth. These potent sensual memories exist in perfect alignment with strong emotional feelings of contentment, safety and love.

We all have sweet memories from childhood—whether it's hot cocoa on a brilliant, icy February afternoon or frozen popsicles melting off the stick in the hot sun of August, birthday cake with ice cream or Thanksgiving pumpkin pie. It's the rare individual whose mental landscape is not dotted with at least some happy memories of sugared moments. So it's not surprising that the urge to replicate these memories (and the feelings associated with them) often carries over into our adult behaviors, whether consciously or not. Because sugary treats are often associated with happy times, many of us may seek out sweets when we are blue. This can become a problem if we start to *need* the taste of sweet for psychological, emotional or physiological reasons.

Is Sugar a Drug?

There's no doubt that everyone requires natural sugars to live and that our attraction to sweet-tasting substances is a biologically important mechanism. Naturally sweet, carbohydrate-based whole foods—such as fruits and berries, starchy root vegetables, even raw honey—have provided humans with energy and nutrients for as long as our species has existed. However, during the past several centuries, the Western diet has seen the addition of sugar and sugar substitutes in forms and levels that were never conceived by nature. And during the past hundred years, the rapidly growing processed-food industry has hooked us on sweets, not just through synthetically intense flavors, colorful packaging and catchy jingles, but also by virtue of the fact that sugar can be physically addictive.

Scientific research has determined that in rats, sucrose stimulates the brain to release dopamine—the feel-good neurotransmitter that activates the reward/addiction pathway. In human studies, sucrose has been suggested to stimulate the release of pain-killing opioids—compounds that bind to receptors in the brain and stimulate the dopamine pathway. All addictive substances and activities activate this pathway. Considering these facts and findings, we may logically conclude that the consumption of sucrose—table sugar—could be chemically addictive.

As many of us know intuitively, both children and adults can easily get hooked on sugar, and research supports this observation. In repeated studies, even babies show a marked preference for sugar-sweetened water over plain water and stop crying quicker when given a sweet drink.

When you combine a built-in biological need for glucose with years of cultural, societal and family reinforcement associating pleasant events with the use of what we now know is an addictive substance, it's no wonder that a weakness for sugar is one of the hardest dietary bad habits to lick.

If you're serious about kicking the sugar habit, switching to natural and healthy sweeteners is one of the best ways to get started.

Sugar's Dark Side: The Bitter Truth

You can't blame an innocent child for sucking on a lollipop. But as health-conscious adults, we know that sugar isn't great for us. On the contrary, sugar consumption can cause or contribute to a host of physical health concerns.

We've already noted how sucrose impacts blood sugar levels and can contribute to insulin resistance, diabetes and related issues—including the rush, followed by the crash, of a sugar-induced blood glucose jolt. But keeping blood sugar in check isn't the only reason to limit sucrose and other high-glycemic sweets.

Obviously, because of its caloric content and metabolic effects, sugar can lead to weight gain and obesity. It also can play a major role in tooth decay, being the favored food of the *Streptococcus mutans* bacteria that live on teeth. Sucrose feeds other bacteria as well, such as the troublesome *Candida albicans* microorganism, which is why high sugar consumption can lead to yeast overgrowth and intestinal dysbiosis (too many bad bacteria).

Sucrose-consuming bacteria excrete a substance called lactic acid. This metabolic process occurs in the mouth and elsewhere in the body where bacteria are found, notably the intestinal tract.

Increased lactic acid and other acids create an acidic, or low pH, environment that may remain local (in the mouth or colon) or become systemic (via the bloodstream). Ultimately, sugar weakens teeth and other bones via the body's response to the effect of sugar on pH balance.

Many natural health experts count sugar as among the most acidifying substances one can consume. (*Please note*: Acidifying foods are those that leave an acid ash after digestion, not necessarily foods that contain citric or other acids. Surprisingly, some seemingly acidic foods like oranges and lemons may actually be alkalizing in the body. Acidifying foods include most grains and flours, coffee and red meat. Alkalizing foods include green tea, most fresh fruits and almost all veggies, especially dark greens and sea vegetables.)

The pH of human blood is tightly regulated to remain between 7.35 and 7.45 (slightly alkaline). Frequent consumption of sugars and other acid-forming foods can drive blood pH into the bottom end of this range, contributing to a state of chronic low-grade metabolic acidosis against which the body must continually defend itself. One method of defense is to pull alkalizing, acid-buffering minerals (calcium, phosphorus, magnesium) into the bloodstream from their primary storage site: bone tissue. This process of "robbing Peter to pay Paul" may succeed in raising blood pH to acceptable levels but it can also lead to bone loss and osteoporosis over time, explaining the link between low bone mineral density and high sugar consumption.

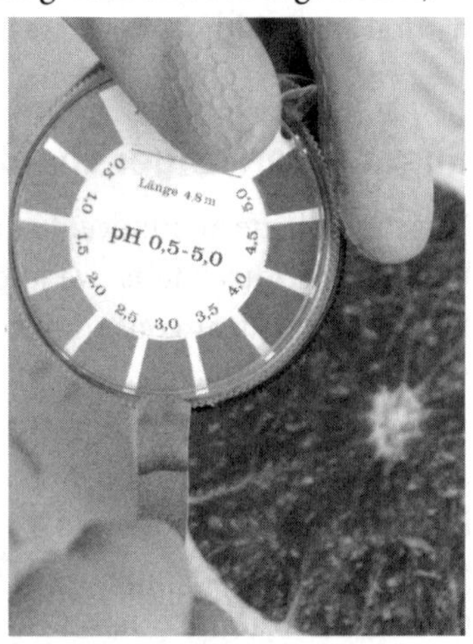

Acidic foods have an alkalizing effect in the body

In addition to teeth and bones, sugar has been long known to weaken the immune system. In one famous experiment from 1976, nutrition pioneer Dr. Emmanuel Cheraskin and colleagues showed that drinking 12 ounces of cola caused a 50 percent reduction in immune-specific white blood cells. In other words, the average 10 teaspoons of sugar contained in one can of soda pop may be capable of temporarily reducing certain immune functions by half. You may have noticed that people who eat a lot of sugar seem to be more prone to colds and illnesses; this explains why.

Considering its effects on immune health, it's not surprising that sugar is a primary food of cancer cells—scary food for thought. And if that weren't enough, consider this: Regular consumption of high-sugar diets has been associated not only with damaging physical effects, but with a long list of adverse psycho-emotional effects as well—from energy imbalances, sleep disturbances and fatigue to anxiety, mood swings, depression and childhood hyperactivity.

See the classic book *Sugar Blues* by William Dufty or more recent works by Dr. Nancy Appleton and others to learn more.

Replacing Sucrose

With all the problems sugar can cause, it's no wonder that people are looking for a replacement. In response, the food industry has identified and brought to market numerous sugar substitutes. Some of these are suitable for use by health-conscious consumers committed to a natural foods diet and lifestyle, others may be more harmful than the original pure sugar itself. For optimum health, we should minimize the use of and need for sweets in general; however, total abstention is an extreme few people require. When a sweetener is called for, natural and healthy options are always best.

Defining *Natural* and *Healthy*

Any discussion of natural and healthy sweeteners calls for a working definition of the word *natural*. (The term *healthy* is self-explanatory.) The U.S. Food and Drug Administration has chosen not to formally define the term *natural*, so there is no legal definition, allowing a broad range of products to be labeled as such.

In the absence of a government guideline, and for the purpose of this booklet, I suggest that to be considered natural or healthy, a sweetener must meet one of the following two criteria:

1. The sweetener is altogether unaltered from the state in which it is found in nature *or* it has been only very slightly altered from this state by use of basic or minimal processing techniques. (Examples are raw honey gathered from beehives in finished form and maple syrup gathered as tree sap and boiled down to syrup.)

2. The sweetener is derived from a whole plant/food source *and* it has a beneficial or benign influence on health. (Examples are xylitol, a tooth-friendly sweetener derived from birch bark, and cellulose, a plant fiber that may be used as a filler or flowing agent in powdered sweeteners like some stevia products.)

Here's what happens when we apply our criteria to pure white cane sugar, which is arguably natural but can hardly be considered healthy:

Pure sugar typically comes from one of two natural plant sources, sugar cane or sugar beets. Both plants—when taken in their natural state—are healthy, mineral-rich foods. When we refine these natural foods through intensive processing, stripping away every trace of fiber and minerals to create a bleached, white crystalline powder, all resemblance to the original food state is lost, along with all healthfulness and nutritional value. Based on commonsense criteria, we therefore do not consider pure sugar to be a natural and healthy sweetener.

Corn sweeteners present a similar situation. Corn is a vegetable that many of us enjoy fresh off the cob in the summertime, either cooked or raw (if you've never tried raw corn on the cob, you're in for a treat—it's like eating candy), and dried year-round (think of cornmeal, cornbread and polenta). Corn kernels, cornmeal and even popcorn are nutritious whole foods containing fiber and other beneficial compounds like eye-friendly lutein and beta-carotene. Highly refined cornstarch and corn syrup made from genetically modified corn are another story.

High Fructose Corn Syrup

High fructose corn syrup (HFCS) is a widely used and, many say, insidiously dangerous sweetener. Since its introduction to the mass market in the 1970s, HFCS has become ubiquitous in processed foods and beverages. Using "fructose" in the name helped sell this product to the American people as a "natural, healthy" sweetener since, as noted earlier, the monosaccharide fructose is naturally found in fruit and honey. However, the FDA revoked the "natural" label claim for HFCS in early 2008.

Pure fructose is a low glycemic sugar that does not significantly increase blood sugar or insulin levels. Potentially, this makes fructose a safe and healthy sweetener, especially for people with hypo- or hyperglycemia and diabetes. In fact, naturally occurring fructose is a healthy sugar for most people when consumed in small amounts as provided by fresh fruit or sensible use of honey, agave or yacón syrup. (The fact that fructose metabolically stimulates fat synthesis is problematic only when fructose is consumed in large quantities.)

But buyer beware! Fructose is not the same thing as high fructose corn syrup, a man-made sweetener derived from cornstarch. HFCS is a concoction made from corn syrup (100 percent glucose) and added fructose.

High fructose corn syrup contains fructose and glucose in approximately equal parts, resembling the disaccharide sucrose. Sucrose consists of bonded fructose-to-glucose molecules. But the fructose and glucose in HFCS are not chemically fused, so the body sees it essentially as predigested sucrose. This means HFCS can enter the system and raise blood glucose and insulin levels even faster than white sugar.

Excess consumption of HFCS has been associated with obesity and high levels of triglycerides and LDL (bad) cholesterol—risk factors for diabetes and cardiovascular disease. Soft drinks are considered a major source of HFCS in the American diet.

Calorie-Free Artificial Sweeteners

Because the number-one reason most people want to eat less sugar is to prevent obesity, the food industry has invested millions of dollars in developing and promoting non-caloric sweeteners. These efforts have resulted in such synthetic sweeteners as cyclamate, saccharin (Sweet'N Low®), aspartame (NutraSweet®, Equal®) and sucralose (Splenda®).

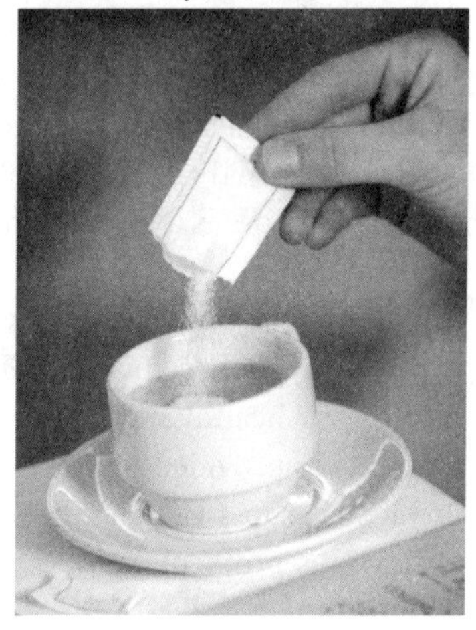

Many sugar substitutes are more harmful than sugar itself.

Despite the food industry's best intentions, none of these artificial sweeteners provide the pure, sweet taste of refined white sugar (or some of the natural sugar alternatives we'll discuss later). Most artificial sweeteners leave a somewhat nasty aftertaste in the mouth. Nevertheless, these products have been successfully marketed and sold to the public. Today, they are a common sight. From lunch counters and rest stops to cafés and fine restaurants nationwide, little pastel packets are everywhere.

If you're trying to lose weight or have a condition like diabetes that requires abstinence from sugar, you understandably may be interested in using non-caloric or low glycemic alternatives. After all, it's natural to like sweets. But if the sweets we like aren't natural and healthy, we may be headed for additional health problems. Let us briefly review four common artificial sweeteners and some concerns associated with each.

Saccharin was accidentally discovered in the late 19th century by a chemist studying coal tar derivatives and first became popular during World War I in the wake of sugar shortages. Saccharin is synthesized from a cocktail of chemicals including chlorine, ammonia and sulfur dioxide. According to the Center for Science in the Public Interest, saccharin is known to cause bladder cancer in rats and has been associated with a similar impact on humans in some epidemiological research. Saccharin is marketed in the United States under the brand name Sweet'N Low®.

Cyclamate was accidentally discovered in 1937 by a graduate student developing an anti-fever medicine. Its taste was found preferable to saccharin, and the product was developed for use as a sweetener in foods and beverages. However, like saccharin, cyclamate has been suggested to increase cancer risk, notably bladder cancer, in animal studies dating back to the 1960s. Cyclamate also may negatively impact male reproductive health and has been banned in the United States since 1969. (Cyclamate is legal in Canada and other countries, where it is frequently combined with saccharin.)

Aspartame (marketed as NutraSweet® and Equal®) was accidentally discovered in 1965 by a chemist developing an antiulcer drug. Considering the controversies surrounding cyclamate and saccharin, newcomer aspartame was welcomed by the diet industry in the 1980s. Unfortunately, it too, has been suggested to cause cancer, notably brain cancer, in lab rats.

Many experts consider aspartame to be a neurotoxin. One product of the breakdown of aspartame, aspartic acid or aspartate, is a known excitotoxin (a class of chemicals that may cause damage to the brain and nervous system), while another, phenylalanine, is forbidden to people with phenylketonuria (PKU), a rare disease that causes mental retardation in the presence of elevated phenylalanine levels. A growing body of additional anecdotal evidence against aspartame can be found on the Internet and in print. Natural medicine practitioners and individuals sometimes report that hard-to-treat issues such as headaches, widespread body pain, menstrual difficulties and dizziness may improve or vanish when people stop consuming aspartame.

Sucralose is the most recent artificial sweetener to hit the market, so less is known about long-term effects. Sucralose was accidentally discovered in the late 20th century by British scientists developing a new pesticide. Marketed as "made from sugar," sucralose is a chemically altered sucrose molecule, synthesized by replacing three of its hydroxyl groups (made of oxygen and hydrogen) with three atoms of chlorine. Chlorine, which is highly toxic to animal life, is a component of bleach and the deadly pesticide DDT. Sucralose is chlorinated sugar.

Marketed as Splenda®, sucralose is 600 times sweeter than refined white sugar. Now found in countless products, sucralose has been suggested in animal research to damage the thymus gland, which plays an important role in immune function. Animal research also suggests that sucralose may raise fecal pH, decreasing levels of beneficial gut flora, which can lead to dysbiosis. Recently, sucralose has been proposed as a migraine trigger in humans. It does not break down in the digestive tract or in nature following excretion, raising environmental concerns as well.

These synthetic chemicals don't belong in our bodies. And table sugar has its own array of issues. Luckily, a wide variety of natural and healthy sweeteners is available to take their place.

Part 2

Natural and Healthy Sweeteners

Now that we understand how the body utilizes sugars and why it's best to avoid refined sucrose and artificial sweeteners, let's take a look at some amazingly healthful natural sweeteners. Starting with agave and ending with yacón, we'll cover a selection of both ancient and innovative sweeteners, available as liquid syrups or dry powders and crystals.

In cases where nutritional values such as calories per serving and glycemic index vary depending on the sweetener's source (e.g., buckwheat or clover blossoms for honey), species, growing climate and production method, a range or average value may be given.

Please be aware that all sweeteners, no matter how natural, should never be used in excess or to replace nutrient-dense, fresh whole foods in the diet. How much is too much? Many health experts suggest that an individual's intake of added sugars should not exceed 40 grams daily. In my opinion, this figure may represent even too generous a helping for regular consumption, considering that one teaspoon of sugar or syrup weighs from four to five grams.

As a holistic clinical nutritionist, I believe that health is best served when we rely upon a plant-based diet of natural, fresh whole foods to nourish body, mind and spirit. That said, there's always room for dessert! To help sweeten up your life, consider the following natural and healthy sweeteners.

Agave Syrup

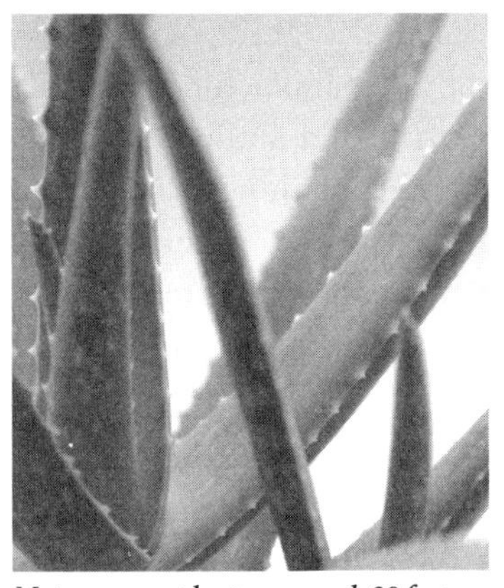

Mature agave plants can reach 20 feet in height.

(*Agave tequilana* Weber cultivar azul, *Agave salmiana*)

Glycemic index: 30–40 (varies with product but always low glycemic)

Calories per teaspoon: 10–20 (varies with product)

Synonyms: organic blue agave, agave nectar

Common forms: clear, pourable syrup; light, amber and dark grades; available in raw form (not heated above 118 degrees)

Features and benefits: low glycemic (diabetic friendly); deliciously pure, sweet taste; mixes easily into liquids; suitable for baking; does not crystallize at room temperature

Agave syrup is one of the newest natural sweeteners in the U.S. marketplace. It arrived near the turn of the 21st century amidst a flurry of exciting health claims and soon earned a place in the kitchen cupboards of many a health-conscious consumer, myself included.

Exotic undercurrents of romance and history embellish agave's appeal. It is made from the juice of a beautiful, succulent plant (related to both lily and amaryllis species) native to Mexico and Central America. Upon maturing, which takes from eight to 15 years, the plant shoots up a gigantic flowering spike that may tower from eight to 20 feet tall.

The flowering agave spike may be severed and a bowl-like hollow carved into the place where the stalk once grew. This causes a sweet, transparent sap, called *agua de miel* (Spanish for "honey water") to seep through the open plant walls and into the hollow. In ancient times, agua de miel was collected and used by the Aztec Indians to make *pulque,* a sacred, traditional fermented beverage. Pulque became the inspiration for another intoxicating drink, tequila, following the 16th-century Spanish invasion of Central America.

Today, most agave for commercial use is grown in Mexico, where the plant has been long used in the manufacture of tequila and mezcal and, more recently, agave syrup and inulin. (Not to be confused with insulin, inulin is a fructose-containing soluble fiber. In agave and other plants such as chicory and yacón, inulin stores carbohydrate energy. In humans, it may function as a prebiotic.)

Agave syrup offers a very pure sweetness, largely unembellished by identifying flavor notes such as those distinguishing maple syrup and honey. Agave can therefore be used to sweeten foods and drinks without altering their flavor, a feature which many tea drinkers and natural food chefs find advantageous. Agave absorbs moisture well, making it great for baking. And it is highly shelf stable, meaning it remains in liquid form and will not harden or crystallize in the bottle as may honey or maple syrup.

Compared to sucrose, agave is one and a half times as sweet and typically contains slightly more calories per serving, hence it is not a diet food. One might argue, though, that since agave is sweeter than sugar, you may consume less of it, leading to a calorie intake of no more than as if you were using sucrose. As a bonus, agave contains small quantities of micronutrients, such as vitamin C, calcium, sodium and iron.

The most significant health feature of agave syrup is that it boasts a very low glycemic index, making it a valuable sweetener for people with blood sugar conditions, such as diabetes, when used in moderation.

Low Glycemic Chemistry and Confusion

Agave syrup contains natural sugars, chiefly fructose, a monosaccharide that does not raise blood sugar levels. The low GI of agave syrup simply results from its high fructose-to-glucose ratio and varies somewhat depending on species and processing method. Agave syrup's naturally high fructose content (ranging from about 50 to 70 percent) may be its top selling point, so it's ironic that, this very feature has led to a degree of confusion in some consumers' minds.

Some people think that since agave is a syrup with a high fructose content, it is equivalent to high fructose corn syrup and is therefore bad. But the agave plant is not and never will be corn, so there is no reason for anyone to jump to this conclusion.

Let's recall that HFCS starts its life as a genetically modified cornstarch, a solid from which is made a liquid—corn syrup (pure glucose)—to which is added free fructose. Agave syrup begins its life as a liquid in the form of the inulin-rich juice of a desert succulent, and stays that way. The fructose that is naturally present in, not added to, agave juice is released during the hydrolysis (breakdown) of inulin, as outlined below. Agave syrup is still processed, yet it is far closer to its natural form than HFCS could ever be.

Remember: Fructose itself is a natural sugar that is healthy for most people, provided it is not consumed in excess through regular use of soft drinks, commercial baked goods, dairy treats and other processed foods containing HFCS. The word *fructose* should not strike fear into the hearts and minds of earnest and informed health seekers.

Agave Syrup Industry Developments

The fledgling agave industry has seen some ups and downs. For example, at least one manufacturer attempted to exploit the syrup's high fructose content by boosting fructose levels even higher. This was allegedly accomplished by spiking agave syrup (some say even with corn syrup, to save on cost) with fructose and other fillers. The result: "agave syrup" with unnaturally high fructose percentages and unnaturally low glycemic index values that are still bandied about, despite their irrelevance. (The company has since folded.)

While such syrups indeed may have been less healthful than properly made organic agave syrups, one bad agave doesn't spoil the whole bunch. Despite intermittently raised concerns about adulteration and integrity, many members of the industry are producing high-quality organic agave syrup in an ethical way.

How Agave Syrup Is Made—Unraveling the Mystery

Several different methods exist for growing, harvesting and processing agave—any of which may be used by the few Mexico-based producers who supply agave syrup to the worldwide market. Due to language and cultural barriers, regulatory inconsistencies and the occasional indulgence in fanciful marketing hyperbole, it can be difficult to ascertain with clarity the exact process used by any given producer.

A few things are certain. Agave syrup does not drip out of the agave plant ready for bottling, nor is it simply the fresh-pressed juice of the succulent. It is a processed natural sweetener, originating from a natural plant source. Agave syrup must be processed, because fresh agave sap (agua de miel) and freshly pressed agave juice both ferment very quickly if not treated in some way (think pulque and tequila).

The age-old method by which agave sap and juice were once processed into a sweetener resembles the way maple syrup is made: slow evaporation-concentration taking place during hours and hours of boiling. It is a simple method that produces a dark, thick, flavorful molasses-like syrup quite unlike the thin, clear, highly pourable agave syrup we know today.

To create the transparent, fructose-rich sweetener that is modern agave syrup, the agave sap or juice must undergo a number of critical steps. These include filtering out impurities (to clarify the syrup) and stimulating the starch-containing inulin molecules naturally present in agave liquids to convert into fructose.

Inulin is converted to fructose by a biochemical process called hydrolysis. Hydrolysis takes place in our bodies every day with the help of enzymes. In the manufacture of agave syrup, hydrolysis may be accomplished in three ways: thermal (application of heat), enzymatic (addition of starch-digesting enzymes) or chemical (addition of strong acids that are later neutralized with caustic soda or lime). Manufacturers of organic agave syrup for the natural products industry should avoid the latter method and instead rely upon thermal or enzymatic hydrolysis.

Agave Syrup from Farm to Bottle

Organic agave farms utilize one of two primary harvesting techniques. On some farms growing the *Agave salmiana* species, the juice may be harvested in the ancient way: removing the flowering stalk from mature agave plants, carving the center into a bowl-like receptacle and gathering the nectar that seeps into the hollow. (One producer claims to practice this labor-intensive method exclusively, having workers collect the sap twice daily from each plant for many months.) On farms growing the more common blue agave species (*Agave tequilana* Weber cultivar azul, beloved by the tequila industry), immature plants are most likely harvested in a different and equally fascinating manner.

First, workers sever the distinctive central spike from immature plants. Normally, this spike would develop into the flowering stalk of a mature plant. Removing the spike drives energy deep into the agave, causing the center to swell into a large, round pineapple-shaped core, also called a heart. These living agave hearts are harvested at their peak of juiciness and transported intact to an agave syrup factory.* At the factory, agave arrives as either liquid sap or in whole core form. In the latter case, cores are cleaned, chopped and pressed to extract the juice within, perhaps being heated prior to chopping to initiate the inulin-to-fructose hydrolysis process. Once the juice is expressed, it undergoes a short series of steps to, again, promote hydrolysis and to remove impurities. Similar steps are applied to agave sap that arrives at the factory already in liquid form.

Depending on the manufacturer, steps in the production of

*Neither harvesting method is recognized as superior, although using the whole-core process seems to address the concern that exposed sap, accumulating for hours in flower-stalk hollows, might be prone to fermentation in the heat of the Mexican sun.

organic agave syrup may include any combination of the following (not necessarily in this order): hydrolysis (by the addition of plant-based enzymes and/or by heating); micro-filtration; evaporation of excess water (by gentle heating, boiling and/or low-temperature vacuum pressure); and purification and clarification of the syrup via ionic exchange. Finally, the finished agave syrup is bottled in-house or shipped in drums to private labelers for packaging at outside facilities.

Producers of "raw" agave syrup claim that all heating takes place below 118 degrees Fahrenheit, the temperature at which enzyme activity in living foods is thought to cease. While this may be true, there are no active enzymes present in any agave syrup. Some suppliers also offer agave syrup in different grades—from light (almost clear) to amber and dark. Darker grades offer a more distinctive flavor.

Enjoy Agave Syrup in Many Ways

Low glycemic agave syrup is a versatile and tasty sweetener. Because it is already in liquid form and readily soluble in water, it's perfect for sweetening beverages. Use it to make "instant" fresh lemonade (half a lemon's juice plus one teaspoon agave syrup per cup of water) or to sweeten coffee, tea and smoothies. Agave can be used in place of honey or maple syrup on pancakes, French toast and nut butter sandwiches, or swirled into yogurt or drizzled on grapefruit. Agave is suitable for baking and is famous in the raw food community for its supporting role in countless scrumptious raw puddings, pies and other uncooked desserts. (Recipes can be found in books and online; try www.goneraw.com and www.thesunnyrawkitchen.blogspot.com.)

However you choose to use agave syrup, always indulge in moderation. Agave is a healthy low glycemic sweetener useful in helping to reduce overall dietary glycemic load, but it still contains sugars (fructose and dextrose) and contributes calories to the diet. Like all nutritive sweeteners, agave will produce fattening, acidifying and other biochemical effects in the body to a degree commensurate with quantity consumed. When consumed in moderation, organic agave syrup is a delicious liquid gift of nature that may be enjoyed by all, including people with blood sugar concerns.

Honey and Raw Honey

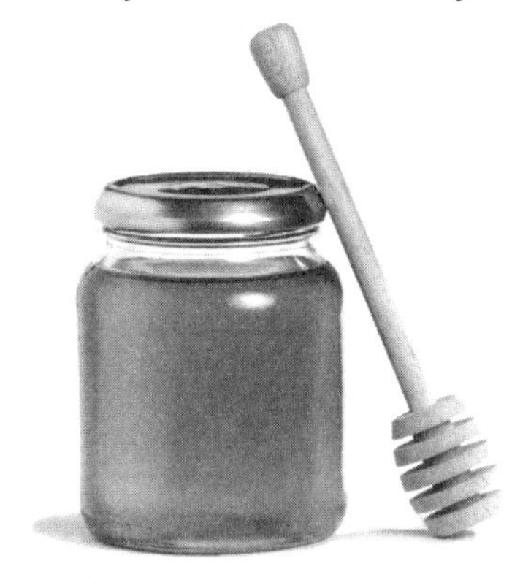

Raw honey contains antioxidants, minerals and antimicrobial enzymes.

Glycemic index: 55 (average; varies with type; see Table 1)
Calories per tablespoon: 64 (average)
Common forms: liquid honey, creamed honey, honeycomb, honey sticks
Features and benefits: highly nutritious—supplies vitamins, minerals and antioxidants; available in many flavor varieties; may crystallize at room temperature; antimicrobial (raw); alive with active enzymes (raw)

Honey, perhaps the original sweetener, is noteworthy as the only liquid sweetener that comes to us in ready-made form, though not always without a price—this golden nectar must be skillfully extracted from the hives of potentially stinging bees. Honey's use dates far back into prehistory. Our ancestors valued it highly and creative methods for obtaining honey have been developed and refined the world over.

Since ancient times, honey has been used not only as food but as medicine. Numerous archaic references suggest honey as a topical dressing for infected areas and to help promote wound healing. Modern research confirms the efficacy of this application, due to the presence of antimicrobial and antioxidant components in raw honey. Studies also support honey's common use as a household remedy for coughs and as an anti-aging skin softener.

A Nutrient-Dense Sweetener

Honey is available in as many varieties as there are species of flowering plants that attract bees. The darker the honey the more flavorful nutritional compounds it contains; lighter-colored honeys are milder in taste. Robust, mahogany-hued buckwheat honey is generally recognized as perhaps the most nutrient-packed variety native to North America.

Nutritious honey contains about twice the calories of sucrose and should be lower in glycemic value, due to its high fructose content. This is why diabetics are sometimes told they may use small amounts of honey from time to time. Findings on the GI of different honeys are extremely variable, however. Australian research reported in the *American Journal of Clinical Nutrition* ranks some raw honey as low as 32 on the GI (glucose scale), with cooked honeys ranging into the 70s and up.

According to USDA data published by the National Honey Board, honey contains several sugars, including 38.5 percent fructose, 31 percent glucose, 7.2 percent maltose and 1.5 percent sucrose, on average. Honey also supplies numerous minerals including 1.3 mg of calcium and 11 mg of potassium per tablespoon, on average, plus phosphorus, sodium, iron, zinc, magnesium, selenium, copper and manganese. Honey contains trace amounts of vitamins C and B, too, along with 18 essential and nonessential amino acids. And it is widely recognized as an outstanding source of cell-protective antioxidant flavonoids and phenolic acids. Honey is more than a sweetener—it's a superfood.

Raw Honey Is Best

Raw honey is filtered and bottled at temperatures below 100 degrees Fahrenheit, consistent with the ambient temperature of the hive. As a living food, raw honey is superior to pasteurized honey. It contains active antimicrobial enzymes, greater amounts of antioxidants and higher nutrient levels. Raw honey may also have a far lower GI than pasteurized honey, helping us to avoid blood glucose spikes and maintain more balanced mood and energy levels. Fresh raw honey is always liquid but often will have crystallized by the time it reaches supermarket shelves. You can re-liquefy any crystallized honey by allowing the jar to sit in a pan of hot water over low heat for some time (make sure it's in a glass jar; plastic can melt). If you are lucky enough to live near beekeepers, you may be able to purchase raw honey directly from the source.

To learn more about this age-old and exceptionally healthy natural sweetener, visit www.honey.org, the Web site of the National Honey Board.

(Caution: Do not feed any type of honey to infants under one year of age, due to the potential presence of bacterial spores that can cause infant botulism. Adults and children over one year of age are routinely exposed to, but normally not affected by, botulism spores.)

Polyols (Sugar Alcohols)

Don't be fooled by the term *sugar alcohols* or put off by the technical-sounding word *polyol.* Polyols are a remarkable class of bulk sweeteners that are sugar free, alcohol free and frequently found in nature—from xylitol in birch bark and corn cobs to erythritol in mushrooms, melons and grapes.

Polyol Basics

Chemically speaking, polyols closely resemble mono- or disaccharide sugars with just a few slight molecular alterations. One notable difference is that polyols contain a hydroxyl (alcohol) group instead of an aldehyde group. The term *sugar alcohol* simply refers to the special molecular structure of these intriguing carbohydrate compounds. (Alcohols occurring as hydroxyl groups are different than ethanol, the intoxicating form of alcohol.)

Polyols are 50 to 100 percent as sweet as sucrose and are sometimes used in combination with each other or unrelated sweeteners (sometimes including artificial sweeteners). Because polyols so closely resemble sugar, they have a similar taste and can often be substituted in equal amounts for sugar when added to foods and beverages.

Fun Facts About Polyol Metabolism

Due to their unique chemical makeup, sugar alcohols are metabolized differently than other carbohydrates. With the exception of erythritol, polyols resist digestion in the small intestine, earning them the title of low-digestible carbohydrates. This means that instead of being absorbed in the small intestine like high-digestible carbohydrates, most polyols travel through the small intestine and into the colon intact, whereupon they are fermented by various types of intestinal bacteria. Some of these gut flora organisms may produce carbon dioxide (CO_2) or fatty acids as a by-product of polyol fermentation.

Intestinal carbon dioxide is, of course, a gas that can be expressed as bloating and flatulence, whereas free fats in the colon may contribute to loose stools. Either of these situations may or may not arise in a given person depending upon individual digestive capability, the type of polyol eaten and how much polyol is consumed at a time. The good news is that, like beans and other low-digestible carbohydrates, polyols have a low impact on blood glucose levels, helping to reduce overall glycemic load. That said, when introducing polyols into your diet, consider starting out with small to moderate amounts in order to comfortably monitor your own personal gut reaction.

Polyol Health Benefits

Overall, polyols offer some fabulous health-related selling points, including a low to very low glycemic effect and an amazing ability to inhibit tooth decay. An additional benefit is that, gram per gram, polyols contain fewer calories than table sugar—sometimes significantly so. And they taste great.

Why Polyols Are So Cool

Another interesting feature of many polyols is that they exhibit something called negative heats of solution, which means energy is required to dissolve the polyol crystals into liquid. This energy comes from heat. So when sugar alcohols dissolve in your mouth, they steal heat from the surrounding oral tissues, causing a temporary reduction in mouth temperature and, consequently, producing a cooling sensation. This effect is more pronounced in polyols such as erythritol, mannitol and sorbitol, and less so in others like maltitol and isomalt. By far, the most cooling sugar alcohol is xylitol, making it a perfect addition to mint-flavored products.

For its refreshingly cool mouthfeel and other reasons, xylitol is one of the most popular and well-researched polyols. To learn more about these useful and fascinating sweeteners, visit the Web site www.polyol.org.

Xylitol

Glycemic index: 7
Calories per serving: 2.4 per gram; 9.6 per teaspoon
Synonyms: birch sugar, wood sugar
Common forms: white crystalline powder
Features and benefits: helps fight tooth decay; provides distinct cooling sensation; less caloric than sugar; low glycemic (diabetic safe); tastes like sugar

Xylitol was discovered in 1891 by the Nobel prize–winning German chemist Emil Fisher during his experiments on xylose, a five-carbon sugar found in hardwood trees and other vegetation. Xylitol exists naturally in many fruits and vegetables, as well as within the human body in small amounts. Originally, it was derived from birch bark and later, corn cobs.

As one of the most popular healthy sweeteners in the natural products industry, xylitol is frequently found as a freestanding bulk sweetener and in sugarless foods, chewable dietary supplements and confectionary and oral care products.

Xylitol Keeps Teeth Healthy

Since the 1970s, hundreds of studies have indicated that xylitol can help decrease the incidence of cavities. *Streptococcus mutans* is an oral-dwelling bacteria that sticks to teeth, feeds on sugars and secretes lactic acid as a by-product. The resulting acidic environment pulls buffering calcium and phosphate salts out of tooth enamel, creating cavities.

Streptococcus mutans can consume polyols such as xylitol, but it can't metabolize them into acids. Instead, sugar alcohols simply accumulate inside *S. mutans* cell walls, weakening the bacteria's ability to function. This helps to explain why sugar alcohols are considered tooth friendly and non-cariogenic: They immobilize oral bacteria.

Most dental research on polyols has been performed using xylitol. Study after study clearly demonstrates that when the typically virulent, cavity-promoting *S. mutans* consumes xylitol, the bacteria's ability to adhere to teeth is inhibited and it cannot grow or reproduce normally. This soon leads to an overall reduction in the total number of mouth microbes and helps maintain healthy oral pH values. The result is stronger, healthier teeth and fewer cavities.

Xylitol's impressive power to help support dental health is why it is found in chewing gums, toothpastes and mouthwashes. Although not yet endorsed by the American Dental Association, several articles attesting to xylitol's benefits have appeared in that organization's official journal. Six grams daily is an amount frequently suggested to help reduce tooth decay; smaller quantities are likely to be preventive.

Xylitol's Other Benefits

The antibacterial benefits of xylitol are not limited to dental health. A recent Boston University study reports that 7.5 to 15 grams daily of a xylitol solution can help reduce the incidence of ear infections in young children. Research from Finland and elsewhere suggests that xylitol may help to block bacteria such as *Streptococcus pneumoniae* from adhering to mucous membranes inside nasal and sinus passageways. Xylitol-containing sinus sprays and nasal washes help provide support for upper respiratory problems. While these products would not be suitable for sweetening your morning cup of tea, they may be of interest to some readers and are worthy of note.

Xylitol is a wonderful, versatile low-calorie and low glycemic sweetener for humans. However, it is not safe for dogs, for whom ingestion of even small amounts can result in vomiting and severe hypoglycemic reactions. (To date, other sugar alcohols have not been found to cause similar adverse reactions in dogs.) Be sure to keep all xylitol-containing products well out of reach of your canine companions.

To learn more about xylitol, see the 2007 booklet *Xylitol: An Amazing Discovery for Health* by Kauko K. Mäkinen, et al., also published by Woodland.

Other Polyols

Glycemic index: ranges from 0 for erythritol to 36 for maltitol powder; from 36 to 54 for maltitol syrups; see Table 1 for details
Calories per gram: from 0.2 to 2.6; see Table 2 for details
Common forms: white crystalline powders and syrups; found in many products
Features and benefits: low glycemic; non-cariogenic (tooth friendly); similar taste and texture as table sugar; low calorie; cooling mouthfeel

Sorbitol was discovered in mountain ash berries by a 19th-century French chemist and has since been found to occur naturally in numerous fruits and berries. Compared to sucrose, sorbitol is 60 percent as sweet and provides about one-third fewer calories. It has enjoyed decades of use as a diabetic-safe sweetener in packaged food products such as cookies and other baked goods. Sorbitol is highly soluble in water and, consequently, highly hygroscopic (absorbs water from the air). Commercially manufactured sorbitol is derived from glucose, typically from corn syrups. High consumption is associated with a laxative effect.

Maltitol is a low-calorie disaccharide polyol that occurs naturally in chicory leaves and roasted malt. Commercially, it may be derived from highly purified corn, potato or sugar beet malt syrups or from cereal starches including corn and wheat, so check with the manufacturer if you are sensitive to any of these foods.

Maltitol is 90 percent as sweet as sucrose—almost equivalent in sweetness to table sugar—and provides only half the calories. As a low-calorie sweetener, maltitol imparts a creamy texture to foods. It is only slightly cooling in the mouth and has replaced sorbitol in some sugarless products, including sugar-free chocolates, because it has a milder laxative effect. Maltitol is the only sugar alcohol available in both dry crystalline powder and liquid syrup forms.

Isomalt is a combination of sorbitol and mannitol. Gram for gram, it has half the sweetness and half the calories of table sugar, with a taste profile almost identical to pure sugar. This is not surprising since isomalt is derived from sucrose.

Like all polyols, isomalt is low glycemic and tooth friendly. Because it does not dissolve easily in water and, concurrently, exhibits low hygroscopicity, isomalt is a prime candidate for use in hard, dry food applications (like sugarless lollipops and cough drops). Along with maltitol above, isomalt is one of the least cooling of the sugar alcohols and, like lactitol below, may function as a prebiotic in the large intestine.

Lactitol was discovered in the 1920s and introduced as a sweetener some 60 years later. Compared to sucrose, lactitol is 40 percent as sweet and provides one-half the calories. Lactitol is noted for having a very pure, clean sweet flavor with no aftertaste. Counter to the reputation of some polyols like sorbitol, lactitol may actually help to enhance gut health. It is digested by healthy probiotic bacteria in the large intestine and therefore functions as a prebiotic. Commercially, lactitol is derived from the disaccharide lactose.

Mannitol is an isomer of sorbitol that occurs naturally in pineapples, sweet potatoes and carrots. Compared to sucrose, mannitol is about half as sweet and contains only one-fourth the calories. Because it does not absorb moisture from the air, mannitol may be useful as a dusting or coating for tablets, candies, etc. Mannitol is derived from specialty glucose syrups and from brown seaweeds such as kelp, a nourishing, fiber-rich marine vegetable. Unfortunately, mannitol's reputation as a laxative exceeds that of sorbitol, so it is probably best used in small amounts.

Erythritol is the only polyol that is readily absorbed by the small intestine. All the other polyols journey through the small intestine and arrive intact in the large intestine, where the bacterial fermentation that may lead to flatulence takes place. But since approximately 95 percent of ingested erythritol is absorbed in the small intestine, only 5 percent makes it to the colon. Therefore, erythritol may be consumed in higher amounts than some other polyols without any noticeable impact on digestion.

Curiously, once erythritol is absorbed by the small intestine it doesn't do much. Like a tourist visiting the body, erythritol quietly enters the bloodstream, is not metabolized in any manner and finally gets excreted via the urine in its original form. The result is that erythritol is completely non-glycemic and supplies less than one calorie per teaspoon, making it the lowest calorie polyol, even though it is nearly as sweet as sucrose.

Erythritol is poorly soluble in water and is non-hygroscopic, making it an ideal sugar alcohol for use in hard, dry food applications like hard candies and chocolates but less appropriate for adding to drinks or moist foods. Commercial erythritol is derived primarily from corn or from sugar cane. It is the only polyol currently available as a certified organic product but not all erythritol is organic; check the label to be sure.

Table 2
Caloric Value and Relative Sweetness of Sugar Alcohols

Sugar alcohol	Calories per gram	Sweetness compared to sugar
Erythritol	0.2	70%
Isomalt	2.0	50%
Lactitol	2.0	40%
Maltitol	2.1	90%
Mannitol	1.6	50%
Sorbitol	2.6	60%
Xylitol	2.4	100%

Note: Sucrose (table sugar) contains four calories per gram or 15 calories per teaspoon.

Stevia

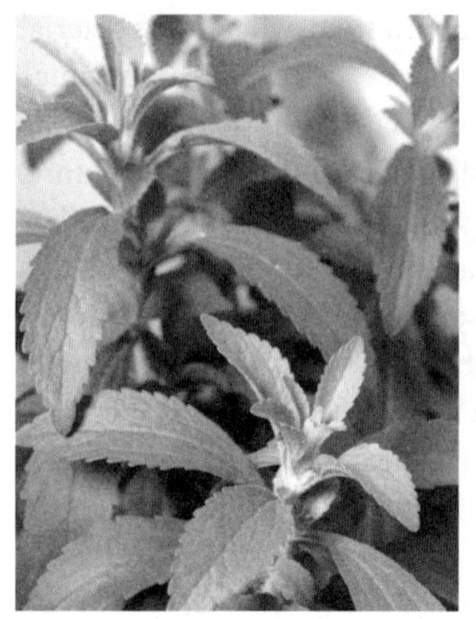

Stevia is available in powdered, crystallized and liquid forms.

(Stevia rebaudiana)
Glycemic index: <1
Calories per serving: 0
Synonyms: sweet herb, sweet leaf, honey leaf
Common forms: whole leaf, powdered leaf, liquid extract, crystalline powder
Features and benefits: calorie free (ideal for weight loss); non-glycemic (safe for diabetics); doesn't promote tooth decay or yeast overgrowth; numerous minerals and antioxidants; suitable for baking

Stevia is a non-toxic shrub that belongs to the aster/chrysanthemum family. Its leaves are extremely sweet, making stevia one of the most unique natural sweeteners.

The stevia plant is native to the high mountain regions of Brazil and Paraguay, where it was first used by ancient indigenous peoples to sweeten traditional beverages such as yerba maté (a tasty and nutritious green tea analog) and bitter medicinal teas. This was accomplished simply by adding a leaf or two of stevia to the other herbs in the pot and allowing them to steep together. Stevia leaves were also traditionally used to help provide digestive support and applied topically as a poultice to help promote normal wound healing.

The Spanish conquistadores discovered stevia in the 16th century and introduced it to Europe at that time, but it took several centuries for stevia to gain commercial popularity around the world. Stevia is currently grown in various South and Central American countries as well as in the United States, Israel, Thailand and China. It is used widely as a sweetener in South America, Japan and Korea and is gradually seeing increased use in North America, both as a stand-alone product and as an additive in low-calorie food and beverage applications. The development of patented stevia-derived sweeteners should greatly increase future consumption in the United States.

For many years, stevia could not be sold as a sweetener in the United States due to a ruling by the FDA. Despite substantial confirmation of its safety, stevia was banned for sale in the United States in 1986, around the time that aspartame came on the market. The total ban continued until 1995, at which time the FDA finally yielded to pressure and permitted stevia to be sold again—under the condition that it be labeled not as a sweetener but as a dietary supplement. This marketing restriction remained in full effect until 2008, when two new stevia extracts were developed and introduced. After reviewing safety studies on these new stevia extracts, the FDA issued letters of "no objection" permitting their use as sweeteners in foods and beverages. In theory, this grants a virtual green light to market stevia as a natural sweetener.

Stevia Components, Research and Health Benefits

Most of the sweetness in stevia is provided by steviosides, glycoside compounds unique to the stevia plant. Steviosides are reportedly 200 to 300 times sweeter than sucrose. Different steviosides may provide distinct sweetness and flavor profiles. One in particular, rebaudioside A, is noted for a very pure sweetness and is the primary component of the new patented stevia extracts.

Stevia also contains high amounts of minerals, notably potassium, calcium, magnesium, phosphorus and sulfur, and significant levels of cell-protective antioxidant phytochemicals including quercetin, apigenin, luteolin and kaempferol.

Stevia and steviosides have been the subjects of extensive research. Safety testing overwhelmingly points to a strong safety profile and supports the claim of nontoxicity. Further research suggests that stevia glycosides may help to support healthy blood pressure and kidney function, may help to fight cavities and may be active against the rotavirus organism that causes diarrhea. Best of all, with its rock-bottom GI value, stevia does not increase blood sugar levels, making it suitable for use by people with hypoglycemia and diabetes.

Stevia in the Marketplace

Powdered stevia and crystallized stevia extracts can be purchased in individual servings and bulk forms that are perfect for sweetening cold and hot drinks, smoothies, salad dressings and desserts. Because of stevia's intense sweetness, very little is needed. Some companies may combine pure stevia with taste-free fillers such as maltodextrin or cellulose to increase total volume and help make stevia usage more familiar or convenient, for example, by allowing you to add a whole packet of stevia to your beverage, rather than just a few grains. Stevia extracts such as rebiana also may be combined with other ingredients or additives. If additives are a concern for you, rest assured that 100 percent stevia powder is available; check labels to know what you're getting.

Stevia is also marketed in liquid extract form, sometimes pre-flavored with essences such as orange or mint. Drops of these liquid stevia extracts may be added to beverages to provide sweetness and flavor, or placed directly on the tongue to help support weight loss by occupying the taste buds and possibly serving as an appetite suppressant.

Finally, you might encounter stevia in bottled or packaged goods, such as pre-made tea drinks or tea blends. For instance, dried stevia leaf may be used in herbal tea bags to enhance flavor and impart sweetness, especially to fruity or medicinal teas. Stevia may also be found in protein powder, hot cocoa and other drink mixes. Expect stevia (and its related extracts) to appear in a host of new products now that the government has allowed this sweetener to be labeled as such.

Stevia: The Bottom Line

Clearly, stevia is a winner on many fronts—especially in the weight-control and blood sugar-balancing sectors. Its only potential downside is that some people may not embrace stevia's distinctive flavor profile, described as being similar to licorice and having a slightly bitter aftertaste. Other folks simply adore the taste of stevia and can't get enough. If you are new to stevia, sample a variety of offerings to find your favorite, as some brands are noted for being more purely sweet than others. The new stevia extract products, which contain added ingredients such as polyols and natural flavors, are another option. As the stevia marketplace expands, more and more people are sure to discover the tasty benefits of this intriguing, unique and remarkably healthy natural sweetener.

Yacón Root

(*Smallanthus sonchifolius*)
Glycemic index: low, no reliable value yet available
Calories per serving: 45 per tablespoon of syrup; 50 per tablespoon of powder
Synonyms: *poire de terre* (pear of the earth), apple of the earth, yacón strawberry
Common forms: thick, dark, flavorful syrup; whole root powder
Features and benefits: low calorie; low glycemic (diabetic friendly); contains prebiotic fructo-oligosaccharides (FOS) to help support intestinal health; minimally processed

Born in the land of Machu Picchu, the high mountain valleys of the Andes, yacón (pronounced ya-CONE) is a tender perennial plant related to both sunflowers and dahlias. Tall and graceful, it sports a long stem topped with small yellow to bright orange daisy-like flowers and is anchored by an underground complex of large, fleshy tuberous roots that resemble sweet potatoes and are noted for their juiciness and incredibly sweet taste.

While technically a vegetable, yacón root is mostly eaten either fresh or dried as a "fruit" in its native Peru and environs, where both roots and leaves have been used as food and medicine for thousands of years. Today, yacón is grown commercially in a handful of South American countries as well as in Japan, Korea and New Zealand.

Although well-known in its Andean homeland, yacón is a newcomer to the North American natural sweetener scene, where its syrup has been heralded in some circles as the new agave. (Both syrups are very low glycemic, but unlike inconspicuously sweet agave, dark brown yacón syrup has a distinct, influential flavor and color, so you may find a place for both in your cupboard.) Also new in the United States is yacón powder for use in baking, desserts and blended foods.

An interesting twist of fate brings yacón to your table. Because it is a poor source of caloric energy, yacón was never highly prized as a staple food by the Incans and their descendents practicing subsistence agriculture under challenging environmental and economic conditions. But it is this very feature that, in part, makes yacón so attractive to modern Western consumers who may desire satisfying low glycemic foods and sweeteners that can complement a sedentary lifestyle without contributing to weight gain.

Low GI Sugars and Healthful Nutrients in Yacón Root

Yacón owes its sweetness to a high content of non-glycemic sugars, notably a subgroup of inulins called fructo-oligosaccharides (FOS). In the body, FOS are not digested or absorbed in the upper digestive tract, so they have no caloric or glycemic impact. FOS arrive intact in the large intestine where they function as a prebiotic, supporting the growth of healthy gut bacteria including the lactobacillus and bifido species. (These healthy flora may help promote immune health through the production of beta glucans.) Depending on time of harvest, up to 67 percent of the sugars in yacón roots are in the form of FOS. Yacón roots also contain lower levels of other sugars (free fructose, glucose and sucrose), numerous antioxidant compounds (chlorogenic, ferulic and caffeic acids), small amounts of B-complex vitamins, vitamins A and C and minerals, such as phosphorus and calcium.

A reliable glycemic index value has not been established for yacón. However, all pure yacón products are low glycemic due to their high FOS content. (Note: Low glycemic products made from yacón root may not raise blood sugar levels but they have never been suggested to lower them, as some may mistakenly believe. This distinction belongs only to the leaf of the yacón plant, brewed as a tea and used traditionally in Brazil to address diabetic, kidney and digestive issues. Yacón leaf extract, but not the root, has exhibited hypoglycemic activity in research conducted on rats with experimentally induced diabetes.)

Special Features of Yacón Syrup and Powder

As with agave, there appears to be no single way to manufacture yacón syrup and powder. Yacón syrup begins as the pressed, concentrated juice of the yacón root. The juice may be boiled down in traditional syrup-making manner or concentrated using low pressure to produce a raw product. In either case, sodium bisulphate or another preservative may be added to prevent enzyme-induced darkening. One supplier (Navitas Naturals) states their yacón syrup is double filtered and flash pasteurized to preserve nutrient content.

Yacón powder is essentially no more than dried, finely ground yacón roots, likely treated in some way to help preserve color and freshness. Yacón powder may be derived from whole yacón pulp, the preservation of which is reported to involve heating to 192 degrees Fahrenheit and adding trace amounts of vitamin C and potassium sulfate to prevent oxidation.

When you are ready to try yacón, be aware of one thing: Because it contains high amounts of low-digestible fiber that passes through the upper GI tract unchanged, yacón may stimulate digestive motility (bowel activity) in some people. A 2008 study at the University of Basel in Switzerland even investigated yacón for its potential role in the treatment of constipation, using generous doses of 20 grams daily with healthy men and women to good effect. For this reason, it's best to start with just a small amount of yacón syrup or powder daily; raise intake gradually as your body adjusts to the increased fiber consumption.

Yacón in Your Kitchen

Thick, luscious yacón syrup has a rich flavor and texture sometimes likened to a mild, fruity molasses. Yacón syrup is delicious spread on nut butter sandwiches or drizzled over hot cereal, pancakes or French toast. It can be baked into pies, melted into caramel sauce or simply used to replace honey or other syrups in any recipe.

Yacón powder is a fine flour-like solid that does not dissolve in water, so it cannot be used to sweeten clear beverages in the same way as stevia and polyols. Instead, yacón powder can replace sugar in baking (substitute equal measure) or be used as an ingénue ingredient in treats like sweet-spiced almonds, chewy fruit bars and puddings. Yacón powder also may be used to enhance the taste and texture of blended soups and drinks, especially those made with rich, creamy ingredients such as banana, raw cacao, coconut and almond milk. Add by the tablespoonful to your favorite shake or smoothie recipe for a glucose-balancing flavor boost.

Let creativity be your guide as you discover the many ways to invent and indulge in exotic yacón cuisine. With a low glycemic impact and flavorful sweet taste, yacón syrup and powder promise to be rising stars in the firmament of natural and healthy sweeteners.

The Sweet Life

The advantages of using natural and healthy sweeteners over refined sugar and artificial sweeteners are well documented. And with so many choices—from flavorful syrups to calorie-free powders—there's surely something for everyone.

In addition to those reviewed in this booklet, other fine and noteworthy healthy liquid sweeteners include 100 percent natural **maple syrup** (a delightful and sustainable forest product originating exclusively from Northeastern U.S. and Canadian maple trees) and grain-based syrups like **brown rice syrup** and **barley malt** (famous in the macrobiotic community for helping to balance the expansive-contractive energies of yin and yang).

Other natural powdered and crystallized sugars include exotic and nutritious **palm sugar** (the evaporated, crystallized nectar of freshly tapped coconut palm flowers), fiber-rich **date sugar** (made from whole, ground dry dates), **maple sugar** (crystallized maple syrup), **sucanat/rapadura** (dehydrated sugar cane juice) and **luo han go** (the dry powdered form of a small, round, intensely sweet gourd in the cucumber family, which is used as a medicinal food in China and tastes similar to stevia).

All of the natural and healthy sweeteners profiled here, and those left unexamined, have their own particular benefits, advantages and preferred uses. May you enjoy exploring their unique offerings and consume them sensibly, in good health always.

References

Barr, R.G., et al. 1999. Differential calming responses to sucrose taste in crying infants with and without colic. *Pediatrics* 103(5):e68.

Bhattacharjee, M., et al. 2005. Antinociceptive effect of sucrose ingestion in the human. *Indian Journal of Physiology and Pharmacology* 49(4):383–94.

CSPI Reports. 10.24.97. http://www.cspinet.org/reports/saccomnt.htm.

Dunayer, E.K. 2004. Hypoglycemia following canine ingestion of xylitol-containing gum. *Veterinary and Human Toxicology* 46(2):87–88.

Foster-Powell, K., et al. 2002. International table of glycemic index and glycemic load values: 2002. *American Journal of Clinical Nutrition* 76(1):5–56.

Geyer, M., et al. 2008. Effect of yacón (*Smallanthus sonchifolius*) on colonic transit time in healthy volunteers. *Digestion* 78(1):30–33.

Ghanta, S., et al. 2007. Oxidative DNA damage preventive activity and antioxidant potential of *Stevia rebaudiana* (Bertoni), a natural sweetener. *Journal of Agriculture and Food Chemistry* 55(26):10962–67.

Hermann, M. and J. Heller, eds. 1997. *Andean roots and tubers: Ahipa, arracacha, maca and yacón. Promoting the conservation and use of underutilized and neglected crops.* Rome, Italy: International Plant Genetic Resources Institute; 223.

Kontiokari, T., et al. 1995. Effect of xylitol on growth of nasopharyngeal bacteria in vitro. *Antimicrobial Agents and Chemotherapy* 39(8):1820–23.

Lotito, S. 2004. Why Apples Are Healthful. *Linus Pauling Institute Research Report.* http://lpi.oregonstate.edu/fw04/apples.html.

National Honey Board. Honey—Health and Therapeutic Qualities. National Honey Board, Longmont, CO.

Ringsdorf, W.M. Jr., Cheraskin, E., et al. 1976. Sucrose, neutrophilic phagocytosis and resistance to disease. *Dental Survey* 52(12):46–48.

Tadhani, M., et al. 2006. Preliminary studies on *Stevia rebaudiana leaves*: proximal composition, mineral analysis and phytochemical screening. *Journal of Medical Science* 6(3):321–26.

Vernacchio, L. et al. 2007. Tolerability of oral xylitol solution in young children: Implications for otitis media prophylaxis. *International Journal of Pediatric Otorhinolaryngology* 71(1):89–94.

Check out these other top-selling Woodland Health Series booklets:

Ask for them by title or ISBN at your neighborhood bookstore or health food store. Call Woodland at (800) 777-BOOK for the store nearest you.

Açaí Berry	978-1-58054-472-6
Alzheimer Disease: A Naturopathic Approach	978-1-58054-423-8
Bee Pollen (2nd ed.)	978-1-58054-429-0
Candida Albicans (2nd ed.)	978-1-58054-432-0
Chelation Therapy (2nd ed.)	978-1-58054-431-3
Chinese Red Yeast Rice (2nd ed.)	978-1-58054-434-4
Coconut Oil	978-1-58054-464-1
Coenzyme Q10	978-1-58054-456-6
Colon Health (2nd ed.)	978-1-58054-435-1
Conjugated Linoleic Acid (2nd ed.)	978-1-58054-433-7
Cranberries	978-1-58054-461-0
Digestive Enzymes (2nd ed.)	978-1-58054-436-8
Fertility: A Naturopathic Approach	978-1-58054-466-5
Fish Oil, Omega-3 and Essential Fatty Acids (2nd ed.)	978-1-58054-437-5
Flaxseed Oil (2nd ed.)	978-1-58054-438-2
Ginkgo Biloba	978-1-88567-010-6
Ginseng	978-1-58054-483-2
Goji Berry	978-1-58054-473-3
Grapefruit Seed Extract (2nd ed.)	978-1-58054-446-7
HPV and Cervical Dysplasia	978-1-58054-463-4
Hoodia (2nd ed.)	978-1-58054-448-1
Hyaluronic Acid	978-1-58054-458-0

About the Author

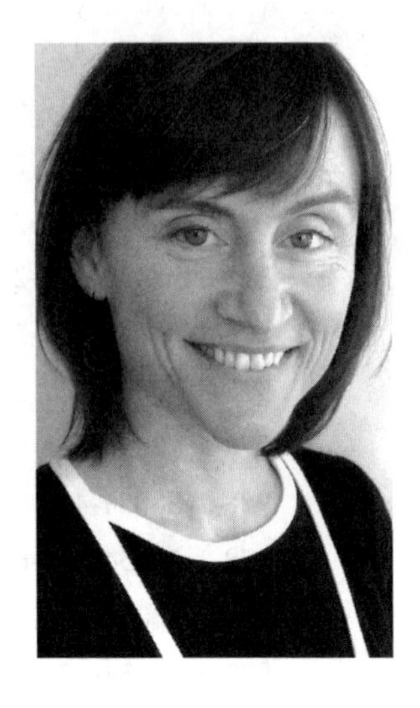

Diana Allen, MS, CNS, is a health writer and holistic clinical nutritionist in private practice in Montague, Massachusetts, where she specializes in food sensitivities, detoxification, traditional whole food diets and raw/living food nutrition. She is the author of numerous brochures and fact sheets for the Pioneer Health Education Library, several articles and the book *Teri Kerr's Ultimate Detox Diet* (with Teri Kerr), published in 2005. To contact Diana, please visit her blog at http://eat2evolve.blogspot.com.